WEIGHT LOSS

How To Lose Weight And Fat Naturally

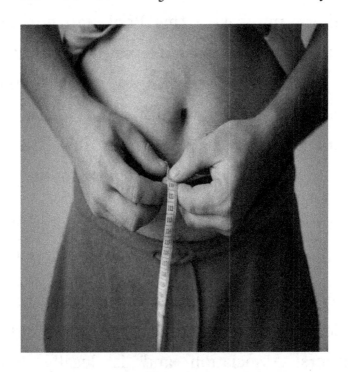

David Scott

considered an endorsement from the trademark holder.

Table of Contents

INTRODUCTION

Most humans have to eat breakfast at some point in the day. According to a lookup done in 2015 using Mintel, a market looking firm, 94% of Americans snack daily. If that percentage is likely to be high-sounding, if you outline a snack as a meal eaten outside breakfast, lunch, or dinner, it is surprisingly simple to notice the last time you once ate. Keep in

Conventional weight loss plan knowledge states that regular snacking is necessary to lose or keep weight. While there is some science to aid the idea, it is tons to show its unnecessary and harmful value. Even dieticians break down on this issue.

Like many nutrition components, there is no simple answer as to whether snacking is appropriate or wrong, but there are some ingredients that can help you figure out whether it will be useful in achieving your goals.

You have probably considered eating 1 to 3 snacks per day between meals a good idea, and logic matters a lot. Anne Danhai, a Scottsdale, Arizona, Scotland, states, "When there is a big-time between meals, your blood sugar decreases, which can make you feel tired, irritable and even give you a headache. Could. " Some humans take the approach of eating 5 to 6 small meals per day to help keep themselves balanced.

"Eating small, standard foods can be especially helpful to anyone who has reactive hypoglycemia or diabetes because of the blood sugar-stabilizing effect," says Danaher. Research has shown that, in particular, high-protein, low-carb, high-fiber snacks are the first in achieving this goal. Additionally, there is Evidence that snacking can help with weight loss, especially in blood sugar issues. One confirmed that high-protein snacks revealed fat loss to patients with type 2 diabetes.

Snacking can also help those who have trouble with component control, Danahy factors out. She explains, "Restraining yourself from being over-starved can benefit someone who struggles with eating temperament because when you do 'hangry' it is challenging to consume your brain and your blood sugar Is destroyed," she explains.

While snacking may help some humans to achieve a healthy eating style, it is honestly not a requirement. "There is a misconception in the world of weight loss plans that you have to eat six small meals per day to lose weight," says Gill, Barkyoumb, MS, RD, founder of Millennial Nutrition. "The science behind this theory is no longer strongly supported. Studies show inconsistent results. "

CHAPTER 1
Switch up your snacks.

Too much snacking can have the opposite effect on your blood sugar. "The more you eat, the more you fill your body with insulin, and the blood sugar fluctuates. This roller-coaster effect on blood sugar can cause cravings, fat storage, and irritability," says Barkyoumb. "To stay away from this, you like to increase your blood sugar levels by using balanced foods with the right amount of protein, fat, and fiber. If your ingredients are balanced and meet your calorie needs, you will no longer want to have snacks between meals since you are genuinely nourished and fueled. "

And although many people cite the idea of "keeping their metabolism jogging at any time of the day," their reasons for snacking do not guide that idea. Snacking is also known to control the urge for food in those who regularly lose weight or keep it. However, according to some studies, the person consuming the snack will receive full energy. Using numbers can have the opposite effect. Days as an alternative to reducing it.

Also, snacking does not allow your body to spoil between meals. "When you're no longer chasing all day, your body has time to digest food and just feel hungry," says Eliza Savage, a CDN at Middleburg Nutrition in NYC. "Yes, it's okay to be hungry!" It is a sign of the body to eat. "She is no longer starving herself," says Key when the snack will probably warrant.

This is why dietitians try to help people determine what a weight loss plan says about enterprise snacking does a high-quality job for them as a person. Danah says, "I like to inspire humans to do a little testing." "Most people have eaten similar methods (and even the same foods) for most of their lives, so I ask them to tune into their bodies and notice that they have unique ingestion patterns and one each. How do you feel about the kind of food? "

Savage agrees, noting that "snacking can be both beneficial and hurt." I think this is the right approach when used correctly and when considering each great and food quantity. I propose strategic snacking, especially at four o'clock. Snack to relieve evening hunger. "She usually suggests making three balanced meals and a snack of protein and a format of vegetables (Hummons, a hard-boiled egg and an apple, a banana and nut butter) for her clients. "Spontaneously, I find that this method is more for humans in weight management phrases with constant ingredients and snacks," she says.

But, at the end of the day, whether you have breakfast or not, it is a non-public option. "More roles in goals, work schedules, food preferences, and the search for the right software for someone," Barkioumb says. That's why snacking - or no longer snacking - is not a requirement for healthy eating for weight loss. You may find it less complicated to take a look at zero snacking to keep your overall calorie consumption down, or you need to eat these snacks more than forests.

Healthy ingredients are extra expensive

It may seem that more healthy ingredients are priced much higher than their unhealthy alternatives. However, if you try to replace components with healthier options, you may find that your elements will work at a lower cost.

For example, choosing cheap cuts of meat and mixing it with more cost-effective preferences such as beans, pulses, and frozen veg would be equally known in casserole or stir-fries.

Carbs put you on weight

Eaten appropriately, and as part of a balanced diet, carbohydrates lead to weight gain on their individual (i.e., they will not be offered except butter, creamy sauces, and so on).

Eat whole grains and whole carbohydrates, such as brown rice and real Bread, eat potatoes with skins to increase fiber intake, and do not eat starchy foods while trying to lose weight.

Starving yourself is the best way to lose weight

Crash diets are not going to result in long-term weight loss. They can gain weight for more extended periods now and again.

The critical problem is that maintaining this weight loss plan is very challenging. You cannot miss essential nutrients as crash diets can be limited in the range of food used. Your body will be low on energy, and you may also crave high fat and high sugar foods. This can lead to eating those foods and more power than you need, which leads to weight gain.

Some foods speed up your metabolism

Metabolism describes all the chemical processes that keep you and your organs functioning internally continuously to function normally, such as breathing, repairing cells, and digesting food. These processes want electricity, and the amount of power required varies between individuals, dependent on elements such as body size, age, sex, and genes.

It is claimed that complementary foods and drinks can increase your metabolism through extra calories and resources, helping the body lose weight. There is little scientific evidence for this. Be aware that some of these products may also contain high levels of caffeine and sugar.

All slimming medicines are preserved to use for weight loss

Not all slimming pills are beneficial or safe for losing weight. There are many prescribed medicines available from your GP for weight loss. Additionally, other un-prescribed, unlicensed weight loss products available on the market may also contain harmful elements for health.

If you are concerned about your weight, seek advice from your GP or any other health care professional.

Constantly low-fat 'or' low-fat 'foods are a consistently healthy option.

Stay alert Foods labeled "low fat" does not have the excess of an excessive amount of fat to use that label legally. If a food is marked as "low fat" or "low fat," it contains less fat than the full-fat version, although this does not automatically make it a healthier option: see Check the label for how fat it is. Are included. Some low-fat foods may consist of high levels of sugar.

Cutting out all the snacks can help you lose weight

Snacking is not a problem when trying to lose weight: it is like a snack.

Many humans need an intermittent breakfast to maintain their power level, especially if they have an energetic lifestyle. Instead of crunchy chocolate and other snacks, choose fruits or vegetables high in sugar, salt, and two fats.

Drinking water helps you lose weight

Water no longer causes you to lose weight, but it keeps you hydrated and may help you have less breakfast. Water is best for precise health and well being. Sometimes thirst can be severe for starvation - if you are thirsty, you can have more breakfast.

Skipping material is an accurate way to lose weight

Content skipping is no longer a fair idea. To lose weight and maintain it, you have to reduce the number of calories you eat and increase the energy you burn through exercise. But skipping foods altogether can lead to exhaustion and may also mean that you release vital nutrients. You will be more likely to snack on high-fat and high-sugar foods, resulting in weight gain.

Does snacking increase your metabolism?

Although it has been recommended that your metabolism will increase every few hours, scientific Evidence will not help.

Research indicates that food frequency has no widespread effect on how much energy you burn.

A person has learned about humans eating the same energy in two or seven ingredients per day; no difference has been found in burning the straw.

In any other study, humans with weight problems confirmed a very low-calorie diet for three weeks, with a relative decrease in metabolic rate, whether they ate 800 calories per day like 1 or 5 ingredients.

Nevertheless, in one study, energetic young men who eat a high-protein or high-carb snack before a mattress have a substantial increase in metabolic charge the next morning.

How snacking effects urge for food and weight

Studies of snacking results on hunger and weight have provided mixed results.

Effect on appetite

Snacking effects urges for food and food intake that is not universally agreed upon.

One assessment stated that although snacks quickly satisfy hunger and promote feelings of fullness, their energy does not compensate for later meals.

This results in better calorie consumption for the day.

For example, in one study, overweight men who eat a 200-calorie snack 2 hours after breakfast consume less energy at lunch.

The ability to increase their calorie intake by about a hundred calories.

In another controlled study, lean people ate three high protein, high fat, or both high carb snacks for six days.

Their starvation and total calorie intake were not unlike those who had not eaten snacks, indicating that they had a neutral effect.

However, research has also proved that snacking can limit hunger.

In one study, men consuming a high-protein, high-fiber snack bar had decreased the starvation hormone ghrelin and high levels of the completion hormone GLP-1. They also consumed an average of 425 fewer calories per day.

Another finding of forty-four girls with weight problems or excess weight suggests that the next morning sleep high in protein or carbs led to decreased appetite and increased fullness feelings. However, insulin levels have additionally been higher.

Based on these results, snacking on hunger depends on the character and type of breakfast.

Effect on weight

Most research suggests that snacking between materials does not affect weight.

Nevertheless, some studies that consume protein-rich, high-fiber snacks may help you lose weight.

For example, a study in 17 people with diabetes noted that an overabundance of snacks on protein and the consumption of slow-digesting carbs reduced weight by 2.2 pounds (1 kg) within four weeks.

On the other hand, some research in obese or normal weight humans has shown that snacking can lead to weight gain or weight gain.

In one study, 36 lean-skinned men increased their calorie intake by 40% using extra energy as a snack between meals. He experienced a full-size increase in liver and abdominal fat.

Some research suggests that snack timing may also affect weight changes.

Finding out about eleven slim girls, it was found out that at 190:00, breakfast of 190 calories. They significantly reduced fat content compared to eating the same snack at 10:00 am.

Mixed-effects suggest that individual and daytime fluctuations lose weight in all likelihood.

Effect on blood sugar

Although many humans believe that it is essential to consume it frequently to maintain stable blood sugar levels throughout the day, this is not consistent.

People with type 2 diabetes find that consuming only two large ingredients per day results in faster blood sugar levels, better insulin sensitivity, and more than ingesting six times per day. Weight is reduced.

Other researchers had noted no difference in blood sugar levels when the same amount of food was fed with the ingredients or ingredients and at breakfast).

Of course, snacks and quant bumps are essential elements that affect blood sugar levels.

Lower-carb, high-fiber snacks have consistently established a more favorable effect on blood sugar and insulin ranges than high-carb snacks in humans with and without diabetes.

Also, snacks with high protein content can improve blood sugar control.

Can there be terrible hunger in the forest

Snacking may not be right for everyone, but it can help some humans avoid being starved badly.

When you go too long without eating, you may become so hungry that you quit consuming many more calories than you need.

Snacking can help make your starvation levels worse, especially when your foods are kept separate.

Tips for healthy snacking

To get the most out of your snacks, follow these guidelines:

Zodiac to eat. In general, it is exceptional to eat snacks that provide you 200 energy and at least 10 grams of protein until the next meal.

Frequency. Your range of snacks varies mainly depending on your exercise phase and food size. If you are very active, you can also choose 2 to 3 snacks per day, while a more sedentary man or woman may again do well with one or a snack.

Portability. Have portable snacks with you when you are on a hunger strike or touring.

Breakfast to avoid. Processed, high-sugar snacks can also provide you with a brief jolt of energy, but you will likely feel hungry after an hour or two.

Our snacking habits

Americans love to snack almost as much as we choose to lose weight. But according to a look through the USDA, our snacking habits include too much energy and too little nutrients. It would not be this way, says Susan Burman, RD, assistant director of the UCLA Center for Human Nutrition. "When done right, (snacking) continues your level of strength and gives you more chances to get all your nutritional requirements."

Eating snacks with the right ratio of nutrients and the right calories will help keep your body active and lose weight. Protein (plus exercise) promotes lean muscle development, which increases the metabolic charge and increases calorie burn. Meanwhile, fiber helps improve digestion and makes you dependent on fats and sugars. So "burn fat" doesn't mean anything until you eat it. As long as you eat it, smart choices with these components will help your body operate most efficiently. Borman suggests under snacks with 10 grams of protein and 5 grams of fiber. Here are 22 of our favorite healthy snacks.

"Almost any fruit is going to make a terrific snack, although you would normally like to combine it with a little protein to make it more satisfying," says Borman; "Unlike carbohydrates, which are imaginatively quickly used, the protein will help maintain your power and appetite levels for a few hours."

Here are some other fruit and diary combo when you crave something rich, creamy, and a little savory. Remove the pit from 1/2 of an avocado and fill the space with 2 ounces of 1% cheese. For 200 calories, you will get 9 grams of protein and 7 grams of fiber - and no dirty dishes!

If you don't want to include dairy in every snack, a can of tuna (packed in water) is another excellent source of lean protein.

For about 200 calories, you can enjoy 3 ounces of light tuna and six whole-wheat crackers - with three grams of fiber and 20 grams of protein.

Lentils are a desirable source of iron, a nutrient that 20% of us do not get enough of. This savory recipe makes four 180-calorie servings, ideal for a hearty, healthy snack. Also, with 10 grams of protein and fiber, it is pleasing to fuel you until your next meal.

Make a batch of white beans and roasted garlic dip at the establishment of the week to spread on the crackers and consume them with starvation when starvation strikes. Serve a quarter cup with 2 cups of raw, chopped cauliflower, for example, eleven grams of protein, 8 grams of fiber, and 199 calories for a whole.

In general, elements that are high in fiber or protein tend to overfill. This ability will make a person feel increasingly satisfied and may consume less in every snack or meal.

Other considerations are finding foods that are low in calories but high in volume or density. The extra house carries a meal in the stomach, the more complete a person can feel. Again, it helps a person eats very little with each breakfast.

People may additionally consider ingredients that aid metabolism and energy. Higher energy can help a person burn extra calories, and a better metabolism can help a character eat food extra effectively.

People searching for weight loss should avoid food that contains large amounts of:

- Salt
- sugar
- Saturated fat
- Simple carbohydrates

Unprocessed ingredients are suitable preferences because many processed snacks contain excessive sugar, salt, or both. Snacking between elements can help with weight loss. Snacking on healthy selection can help to supply vitamins, fiber, and protein to anyone.

The following are some of the first-class snacks for weight loss.

1. Hummus and Vegetables

Hummus is a classic Mediterranean dish made from pure human chickpeas. Due to its developing popularity, shops often have a variety of flavor options for premature hummus dips. People can additionally make hummus at home.

According to a 2016 study source, hummus offers many appreciable benefits. The hummus presents a top protein and fiber source, which can help a faster fuller.

When people consume hummus with vegetables, they also benefit from humus and extra nutrients from vegetables.

2. Celery Sticks and Walnut Butter

Celery is a low-calorie vegetable. According to the United States Department of Agriculture (USDA), two large celery stalks depend on 2.5 cups per day for a 2,000-cup diet as 1 cup of the integral.

Celery is especially water, which can help a person feel full. Dipping celery in nut butter, such as peanuts or almond butter, may supply the benefits of healthy fats and proteins.

3. Fruit and Walnut Butter

Apple and peanut butter is a convenient diet-friendly snack.

People can get creative with their fruit and nut butter mixture if they wish. According to the USDA, a medium apple provides 20 percent of a person's dietary fiber and supports 1 in 2 fruits per day.

Dipping an apple piece in peanut or every other nut butter adds protein and precise fat to a person's breakfast.

4. Low Fat Cheese

Low-fat cheese wares offer many nutrients and reduce fat content compared to everyday cheese.

Some of the benefits include:

- Source of protein
- Source of calcium
- Source of various nutritional vitamins and minerals

- Low-fat cheese also has fewer calories than full-fat cheese.

5. Nuts

Nuts can be a very healthy and filling snack.

Nuts provide protein and the right fat. However, to ban their salt intake, these people took a look at the label to say that there is no complimentary salt. A person should also stay away from nuts cooked with flavors, noting that the flavors regularly contain sugar or salt.

Instead, people should eat uncooked or dry-roasted nuts. Nuts are high in calories, so a person has to eat small amounts per snack.

6. Hard-Boiled Eggs

Eggs are a tremendous source of protein. However, in previous years, many people think that eggs are no longer healthy due to cholesterol concerns.

However, recent additional research suggests that eggs do not increase LDL cholesterol and include many essential nutrients.

7. Greek Yogurt with Berries

Greek yogurt is high in protein and calcium and low in fat and calories. A man or woman can safely add sparkling fruits or nuts to Greek yogurt to improve their style and adds value to the diet.

First-rate Greek yogurt is a straightforward variety of weight loss. Greek yogurt with flavors will often include more sugar, which is no longer desirable for weight loss.

8. Adame

Gamay is a legume that a person can consume for breakfast. Like other legumes, edamame is a supply of fiber and protein.

It is also high in potassium, iron, and magnesium. When humans eat it between meals, edamame can help a person feel fuller while also supplying essential nutrients.

9. Air-popped Popcorn

Popcorn is a famous snack food in America. It is often poorly recognized because of the added sugar, fat, or salt that humans put on it.

Air-popped popcorn does not include these additional ingredients. Plain popcorn is a low-calorie full-grain that presents a lot of filling fiber.

Eating a snack between the ingredients helps curb your appetite so that you sooner or later take a seat to eat. Snacking can also help you get all the vitamins you need. On the flip side, grazing on food throughout the day — especially those with little dietary value — can lead to too much consumption. It is a remarkable notion to have snacks at the grocery store and pack them for work, so you are ready when you go on a hunger strike. Many of these are also tremendous on snack options.

Can snacking be part of a nutritious diet? For sure! When you take out a snack, take out one with protein, fat, and fiber. All these nutrients take longer to digest, so they fill you up. Snacks are a great way to add more vitamins to your day. Think of snacks like carrots and hummus, an apple with almond butter, or whole-grain crackers with cheese.

What about breakfast?

The biggest problem with hour-long dark snacks is that most of us reach ice cream and chips — not fruits and yogurt.

This is to say that you can no longer treat after dinner. Some of your favorite nighttime snacks may also be on this list (chocolate! Popcorn!).

One element to note is that if you are frequently hungry after dinner, make positive that your food is filled with filling and healthy foods and getting enough food.

If you are nibbling on everything, then there is a crunchy salad that you can legitimately starve and want a night snack (see our Extraordinary Dinner for Weight Loss). If you prefer dinner after dinner, serve yourself a healthy element in a plate or bowl so that you are no longer scooping directly from the container.

1. Almonds

Nuts are a first-rate nutritious snack. And even though they are high in fat, if you are trying to lose weight, you do not want to avoid them. One study has found that people who chewed almonds thoroughly (up to forty chews) feel longer than those who chew nuts in small amounts. Also, almonds supply fiber, protein, and healthy fats.

An almond, one ounce, or 23 almond serving contains 164 calories, four grams of fiber, and 6 grams of protein.

2. Grapefruit

You do not want to go on a grape diet to get this ruby fruit's fitness benefits. A whole grape has about one hundred energy and 4 grams of fiber. Not to mention, it saves one hundred percent of women's diet C for the day. This spicy citrus fruit has a lot of nutrition (see different powerful health objectives for eating extra grapes).

One has found that when humans eat grapes clearly with every meal, they lose up to 3 pounds in three months. Researchers say that grapes can help control hunger by reducing insulin levels.

3. Chiku

Put chickpeas in the panties. When you're gaining weight, they have a creamy texture and a nut-like flavor, with plenty of saturating fibers and little protein-rich. Try roasting them for crunchy breakfasts that pack quickly.

1/2 cup of chickpeas has about one hundred calories, 5 grams of protein, and 5 grams of fiber.

4. Grapes

Toss the grapes for a simple snack in the freezer. Because they are sweet and you appreciate them personally and slowly, you can get plenty of pleasure for just a handful of calories.

Even though grapes have a high sugar content for fruits (see our rating of fruits from lowest to absolute best carb), they are a high-quality way to satisfy your sweet tooth naturally. One cup of grapes contains about a hundred calories.

5. Chocolate

Losing weight does not suggest giving up the foods you love. Believe it or not, giving your small treats can also be the secret to losing weight - suitable for. Aiming to thwart "excellent" units does not allow you to have complete revelations in your foods.

If you like a glass of wine with dinner, make room for it. Do you like sweets? Skip the drink and go for a small chocolate treat instead. Remember, if you have both, this is fine. Do not beat yourself up. Enjoy nutritious breakfast tomorrow.

6. Popcorn

Popcorn is high in fiber and may provide even a little protein. A 1-ounce (about 3 cups) air-popped popcorn contains 4 grams of fiber, about four grams of protein, and one hundred and ten calories. This mixture of staying power makes it a snack. Popcorn is honestly a whole grain, and 3 cups is a huge serving — primarily when you evaluate it with other crunchy, salty snack chips. Many agencies are making brinjal popcorn; see our favorite healthy popcorn pics.

7. Yogurt

Use snacks to fill dietary gaps. Choose those that supply calcium and fiber — two vitamins that humans regularly skimp. Yogurt with fruit distributes calcium and fiber, plus protein and gut-healthy probiotics.

Choose simple yogurt and add your fruits for natural sweetness and fiber. Delicious yogurt often promises lots of sugar and more calories. Whole milk and low-fat waterless yogurt are also healthy options. New lookups on dairy have debated the fab that fat-free is healthy.

8. Hummus

Leave the merchandising computer and satisfy lunch with the "healthy breakfast" that you packed at home. You will save money and make a big bang for your nutritional buck. Try to reduce the number of veggies and some hummus. A serving of hummus is two tablespoons.

Planned snacks that offer both complex carbohydrates and protein will help you tide over until dinner. Learn more about the fitness benefits of hummus.

9. Oatmeal

Oatmeal is a complex carb, which means that it replenishes you and increases your blood sugar. Also, it is an accurate supply of fiber, and the intake of excess fiber helps people lose weight and keep it off. While we usually think of it as breakfast, a small bowl of oats makes for a hearty, filling, and delicious snack. To make this snack more convenient, place a packet or two unsweetened instant oatmeal on your desk or make oats in a single day in a mason jar.

10. Dry Fruits

Dried fruit is a portable, nutritious snack. Eating fruit helps to lose weight, as it is packed with fiber (and essential nutritional vitamins and minerals). Look for fruits with no sugar or sweeteners and add dried fruits with nuts to snack with nutritious carbs and protein consistency. Dried fruits are also an excellent option to preserve at your desk at work.

If you are trying to lose weight, then snacks can be healthy in your weight loss program. Thinking about nutritious snacks to pack for work snacks, snacks to snack on, store-bought snacks, and snacks you can make yourself will help you separate the vitamins that will help you between meals. Prevents hangs. Remember, consuming nutrient-rich (fiber, protein, vitamins, minerals) and snacks will help you meet your body's needs and give you complete protection.

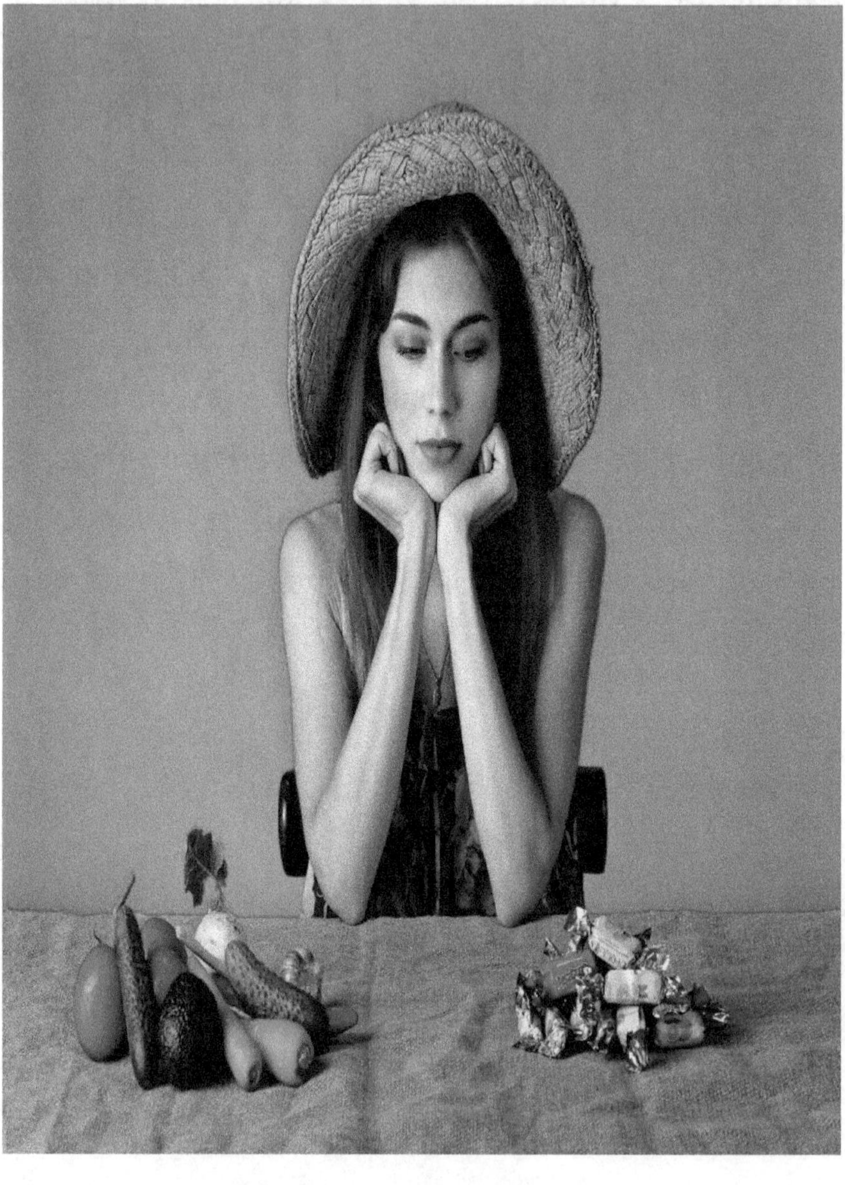

CHAPTER 2
Cut out high-calorie condiments and sugars

Traditionally, when we infer spices, we consider mayo and mustard - they are standard, classic sandwich toppers. Today, spice options are a terrible lot stronger. Plenty of flavored mustard to barbecue sauces, the selections are enjoyable and potentially confusing. In addition to toppers, spices are used to marinate for cooking, tenderize proteins, enhance flavor, and add a palate charm.

Although most spices are not given many vitamins in your diet, some contain healthy ingredients such as herbs, spices, heart-healthy fats, and antioxidants. Whether you take out healthy or healthy-healthy spices, it is usually brilliant not to drown your food. Instead, stick to the serving size. two

Healthy Spices to Add to Your Food

Spices that make it to the healthiest list are low in calories and unhealthy fats and are made with quality, much less processed substances that incorporate fitness benefits.

Mustard

Mustard is a very low calorie (only five energy in a spoon), carbohydrate, and fat-free spice that can enhance food taste by adding a spicy kick. Most of the standard mustard, both yellow and spicy, are made from distilled vinegar, garlic powder, mustard seeds, onion powder, salt, spices, and turmeric. This ability mustard incorporates negligible calories, fat, protein, and carbohydrates in one serving.

Also, studies have proven that turmeric can have health benefits. Turmeric contains a compound called curcumin. Preclinical studies advocate that curcumin can act as an antioxidant and has anti-inflammatory, anticancer, and neuroprotective properties. Therefore, aromatic mustard such as honey mustard can be introduced, making it positive to read the label continuously before eating.

The following nutrition records are provided using the USDA for one teaspoon pickled mustard.

- Calories: 5
- Fat: 0g
- Sodium: 50 mg
- Carbohydrate: 0g
- Fiber: 0g
- Sugar: 0g
- Protein: 0g

vinegar

Whether balsamic, white wine, or apple cider, vinegar can be used for top sandwiches, gown salads, facial dishes, and Marinette foods. This spice is calorie-less (from 0 calories to 10 energy per teaspoon) and contains no sodium. Studies have proven that apple cider vinegar, in particular, can limit fasting blood sugar in humans who are at risk for type 2 diabetes.

Hot sauce

The hot sauce, which includes the original Tabasco and Sriracha sauce, is made from red chili peppers, which gives it a spicy flavor. Adding spice to your food can saturate it and help reduce your hunger and speed up your metabolism. Read the label before pouring, as Sriracha may contain sugar. Try your cereal scramble, vegetables, or whole grains with a sprint of hot cereal.

Pico de Gallo

This low calorie, low fat, delicious and nutrient-dense salsa can zest any meal. Traditionally made with tomatoes, onions, jalapeno, and lime, you can easily make your retailer on sodium. Top your salads, vegetables, or protein with this to add flavor. Or, simply dip it as fresh, raw greens as breakfast.

sauce

It was a tablespoon containing 20 calories, 5 grams of sugar, and 4 grams of carbohydrate in a spoon. Due to its carbohydrate and sugar content, ketchup is a spice that wants to be partially controlled, mainly for humans with diabetes following a modified carbohydrate diet.

However, if you can stick to a portion and remove a type of ketchup that is not made with excessive fructose corn syrup, it can be blanketed in a nutritious meal plan, mainly if you are looking for a creamy look. High-calorie items are changed into dressings or buttercreams.

Unhealthy spice alternatives

Gadgets from the unhealthy pick out the list are high in calories, sodium, fat, and sugar for a short serving. If you repeatedly use these gadgets, you may wish to cut the low back and try to replace them with spice in the entire list.

Creamy Salad Dressing

The creamy salad dressing is made with sugar, bitter cream, mayonnaise, and egg yolk, rich in calories, sugar, and saturated fat. A small serving can handle a ton of calories.

For example, two tablespoons store-bought creamy Caesar dressing contains one hundred and seventy energy and 18 grams of fat instead of 90 life and 9 grams of fat compared to a vinaigrette dressing.

Mayonnaise

The primary purpose of this list is mayonnaise. This is since it is exceptionally high in energy for a small fraction. Although it is made up of complete substances such as egg yolk, olive oil, and vinegar, a tablespoon of mayonnaise can cost you a hundred calories and 11 grams of fat. And while it is unsaturated (complete type) of great fat, it can be challenging to manage this spice, leading to excess calories.

If you are searching to control your weight, mayonnaise is a simple ingredient to remember from your meals to reduce your universal calorie intake. When topping the sandwich, replace the mayonnaise and use a small amount of avocado or hummus as an alternative to making tuna or egg salad.

Barbecue sauce

Barbecue sauce is moderate in calories, with about 60 in two tablespoons, although it also contains a considerable amount of sodium and sugar in one serving. Most manufacturers have about 10 to thirteen grams of sugar (equivalent to three teaspoons of sugar) and 280 to 350 milligrams of sodium.

Another issue with barbecue sauce is that most people do not follow the serving size, two tablespoons. Therefore, if you are trying to look at your calories and sugar consumption and use barbecue sauce, the goal will be to serve one.

Added sugar, such as desk sugar, honey, and syrup, should not exceed 5% of the strength you get from eating and drinking each day. It is about 30 grams a day for people 11 and older.

Many expressions of sugar

There are loads in different ways. Sugar can be listed on the components label:

- Sucrose
- Sugar
- Fructose
- Maltose
- Fruit Juice
- Jaggery
- Hydrolyzed starch
- invert sugar
- corn syrup
- Honey

Nutrition labels tell you how much sugar is in the food:

High in sugar - 22.5 grams or more sugar per 100 grams

Low in sugar - 5g or less than 100g of total sugar

Some packaging uses a color-coded machine that makes it easier to select low sugar, salt, and fat. Look for more "greens" and "amber" in your shopping cart and less "red."

Breakfast

Many breakfast bowls of cereal are high in sugar. Try switching to low-sugar grains or those with no added sugar, such as:

- Plain porridge
- Plain whole grain biscuits
- Plain chopped whole pillows

Swapping a sugar bowl for a simple breakfast cereal can reduce your diet plan by 70 grams of sugar (up to 22 sugar cubes) a week.

Oatmeal oats are low-cost and contain vitamins, minerals, and fiber. Make oatmeal with semi-skimmed, 1% or skimmed milk, or water.

If you usually add sugar to your oatmeal, try adding chopped dried apricots or a sliced or mashed banana instead. Or you should try our apple-pie porridge recipe.

You can eat sugar grains and simple grains on alternate days or mix each in a single bowl for a more gradual approach.

If you add sugar to your cereal, you should try including less. Or you can eat a small element and add some chopped fruit, such as pear or banana, which is a simple way to get some of your 5A Day.

Read our guide to choosing nutritious breakfast cereals.

If toast is your breakfast staple, try whole or chickpea Bread, which is higher in fiber than white bread, and see if you get less help with your traditional spread like jam, jam, honey, or chocolate can do. Or you should try the sugar-free or low-sugar option.

main course

Many meals that we do not reflect on consolidation for candy contain an enormous vast amount of sugar. Some prepared soups, stir-in sauces, and ready meals may also have more sugar than you think.

1/3 (about 150g) of an average-sized jar of pasta sauce can contain more than 13g of sugar with the dispensed sugar - the equivalent of 3 tablespoons of sugar.

When consuming or purchasing a takeaway, usually look for high sugar dishes, such as sugar and sour dishes, candy chili dishes and some curry sauces, salads with dressing like salad cream, which is also excessive in sugar Cans.

Spices and sauces like ketchup can contain 23g sugar in 100g - about half a teaspoon per serving. These foods are usually served in small amounts, although they may depend on sugar if eaten each day.

Takeaway Get directions on making healthy choices when buying food and eating out.

Snacks

Healthy snack options include sugar brought in, such as fruit (fresh, tinned, or frozen), unsalted nuts, unsalted rice cakes, oatcakes, or self-made plain popcorn.

If you are not ready to give up your favorite flavors, you should start by getting less. Instead of 2 biscuits in 1 meeting, try to be 1. If you have two times in your snack, share one and the other, or retail it for another day.

If you are an "all-and-nothing" kind of person, you want to do something to remove your idea from food on certain days of the week.

While shopping, reach out for low-sugar (and low-fat) versions of your favorite snacks. Buy small packs, or bypass family items and go for an average size instead.

Here are some low-calorie options for popular snacks:

Cereal bars - Despite their healthy image, many cereal bars can be excessive in sugar and fat. Watch out for bars that are low in sugar, fat, and salt. Or try this fruit granola bar recipe to make your own.

Chocolate - Swap for a low-calorie hot instant chocolate drink. You can additionally get chocolate with coffee and chocolate with malt varieties.

Biscuits - Swap for oatmeal, oat biscuits, or unsalted rice cakes, which also give fiber.

Cake - Swap for a simple currant bun, fruit scones, or malt loaf. If you add toppings or spreads, use them sparingly or choose low-fat and low-sugar varieties.

Dried fruits, such as raisins, dates, and apricots, are high in sugar and can be severe for your dental health as it sticks to your teeth.

To prevent tooth decay, dried fruit is preferred at mealtimes - as a dessert stage, for example - rather than breakfast.

The drink

About a quarter of the distributed sugars in our diet come from sugary drinks, such as fizzy drinks, sweet juices, squash, and cordials.

A 500 ml bottle of cola contains 17 cubes of sugar. Try sugar-free varieties with a splash of fruit juice, or - more but water, low-fat milk, or soda water.

If you take sugar in tea or coffee, regularly limit the quantity until you can cut it completely, or try swapping the sweetness instead. Try some new flavors with natural tea, or make your lot with warm water and a slice of lemon or ginger.

Like some fizzy drinks, fruit juice may be high in sugar. When the liquid is extracted from the entire fruit to make fruit juice, the sugar comes out, and this can damage your teeth.

Your blended drinks with fruit juice, vegetable juice, and smoothies should not drink more than 150ml a day - which is a small glass. For example, if you have 150ml orange juice and 150ml smoothie in a day, you would have submitted the recommendation through 150ml.

Fruit juices and smoothies contain vitamins and minerals and can count towards your 5A day. However, they can at any time depend on a maximum of 1 part of your 5A day. For example, if you have two fruit juice glasses and one smoothie in 1 day, it only counts as 1 part.

You may want to try flavored water with a slice of lemon, lime, or fruit juice. But look out for the sugar content in the aromatic water drink: a 500ml glass from some manufacturers contains 15 grams of sugar - about four teaspoons of sugar.

Sweet

Work on some ground rules. Do you need dessert every day? How about dessert entirely after your dinner, or dessert only on the bizarre days of the month, or only on weekends, or only in restaurants?

Should you have chocolate, biscuits, and cake each day? If you have this type of sugary snack very rarely, would you like it more?

Low-sugar muffins include fresh, frozen, dried, or tinned fruits, but choose those canned juices as an alternative to syrup - such as low-fat and low-sugar rice pudding and direct low—fat curd.

However, fat reduction does not mean low sugar. Some low-fat yogurts can be sweetened with refined sugar, focusing on fruit juices, glucose, and fructose syrup.

If you are stuck between choosing two cakes in the supermarket, why not evaluate the labels on each of the programs and go with the number of sugar shortages for 1.

Nothing is more frustrating than watching your weight, even if sticking to the round lean protein, veggies, and whole-grain building ingredients. The problem should be sauces, spreaders, and dips you add to any other health food. No one needs to eat Bland food, but the spices we use in our ingredients are regularly filled with sodium, sugar, fat, and preservatives. With just a few grinds or molasses, your nutritious food can be ruined.

The trick is finding out which people are thwarting your efforts to consume better. Some are obvious; others are a bit sneaky. Fortunately, we have completed research to reveal the 15 spices you need to avoid. An occasional spread is fine, but keeping these additions from your fridge will go a long way towards increasing your diet.

1. Ketchup

Everyone's favorite French fry dip sounds like a decent wish - it's made with tomatoes. The sad truth is that this spice is full of sodium and sugar. Eating a tablespoon will get you back to 167 milligrams of sodium and 3.4 grams of sugar, and most of us are using way more than that small portion.

Men's Journal warns ketchup that you should aim to consume extra than you in any other case, which can make matters worse. For a healthier option, try your favorite food, including salsa. It is in full flavor except for all added sugar and sodium. You can also make your very own with a squeeze of tomato, onion, garlic, jalapeño, cilantro, and lime.

2. Sricharan

No hot sauce meets Sriracharya's form of love. There is even a cookbook full of things that you can prepare dinner with Sriracha. Since they are low in calories, hot sauces catch applause, but the energy is not entirely different when a spice is off the charts in various nutrients. One tablespoon contains eighty milligrams of sodium.

Also, it does not provide a very high nutritional value - and too much hot sauce intake can harm you.

Hot sauces like Sriracha are exceptionally acidic, which can cause stomach ache. According to Livestrong.com, capsaicin is found in hot peppers and is used in condiments like Sriracha, which can irritate your stomach's lining if you consume it in plenty.

And while Sriraka will likely not cause digestive disorders, it can flare up in humans who already have them. Cooking with clean hot chili to add a little spice to your meal is a first-class way to reduce your sodium intake.

3. Ranch Dressing

If you explore one aspect of the farm with your order eating whole, you are no longer alone. But this is a risky item - a tablespoon of poppy contains seventy-three calories, about 8 grams of fat, and 122 milligrams of sodium. Once again, large component sizes can do considerable damage. When you order dressing favors at a restaurant, it usually comes in a rake of about 2.5 ounces, with five tablespoons of the ranch. This is the energy of almost perfect food that you include in your salad or entree.

If you crave a creamy dip, try similarly cooking some Greek yogurt. A little minced garlic, some chopped dill and parsley, a dollop of hot sauce, and some pepper will fundamentally turn into that delicious topping.

4. Barbecue Sauce

Grilling is an innovative strategy to make a nutritious meal loaded with flavor if you do it correctly. Sadly, two tablespoons of fashionable barbecue sauce contain about 60 energy and 13 grams of sugar. Since the American Heart Association recommends limiting their consumption of sweet stuff, no more than nine teaspoons a day for men and no more than six teaspoons for women. Consuming this sweet, spicy sauce can send you to that point without any difficulty.

For a topical treatment, making cookout seasoning at home is a healthy option. One serving of The New York Times barbecue sauce recipe is just 45 energy with three grams of sugar. You can additionally add flavor to your protein and add a pickle. Try to use substances like garlic, lemon, and fresh herbs to taste except for all the sinister stuff.

5. Horseradish Sauce

Horseradish sauce is often served with meat or fish or as a section of shrimp cocktail sauce. This provides a spicy kick to something that you fill with it, although it is not a taboo cost. The majority of calories serving a single teaspoon of horseradish come from saturated fat. If you eat it low in fat and something, then this probability will not be so high. But this is no longer the case with beef or seafood.

Dietary Guidelines for Americans recommend not consuming more than 10% of each day's excess energy from saturated fat. Just one tablespoon of horseradish sauce produces about 2 grams of saturated fat, which can start adding to you when you are generous with your portion; for a more healthy way to decorate your food, decide on herbs and spices.

6. Light Salad Dressing

Bottled salad dressing is never an exact desire for mediocre style and has a remarkable price charge tag. Surprisingly, excessive fat content should be less than your concerns. Dr. X pointed out that removing the fat from the salad dressing capacity requires changing it through sugar and different additives to achieve the same texture and taste. However, the enemy is not the enemy. A little oil is desirable to incorporate with greens only since it allows you to absorb fat-soluble vitamins.

Skip the pretense stuff and make your own. As long as you have vinegar or citrus, some nutritious cooking oil, and some seasonings, you can do it together in a few seconds.

7. Cream Cheese

Bagels are not the best breakfast option, although you can make carb-heavy meals very healthy to choose whole wheat. Despite this, if you are leaving it with a lot of cream stuff, you will be in trouble. A typical unfolding serving in Panera Bread is four tablespoons, which will add one hundred ninety calories and 18 grams of fat to your bagel.

The exact news is that you have lots of delicious options that are very healthy. If you crave some type of creamy dairy, you can spread to ricotta for fewer calories, less fat, and more protein. Other precise selections include hummus, nut butter, and mashed avocado.

8. Mayonnaise

This creamy spread makes it much better than any sandwich style, although it comes at a cost. Made from whole eggs and oil, it is about 100% fat. And won't be fooled through restaurants that use the word restaurant. It is the same ingredient with garlic, olive oil, and perhaps a few different flavors.

Try to use a small amount of spread when making sandwiches. You can also pull it with the help of mixing in some mustard, herbs, or chopped vegetables. Greek yogurt is any other exceptional option, and many tuna and rooster salad recipes use it to remarkable effect.

9. Soy Sauce

Unlike other preferences on this list, soy sauce is low in calories, fat, and sugar. The trouble with this Asian staple is sodium. While proper seasoning is a reasonable way to ensure a tasty meal without adding tons of different ingredients, it is simple to go overboard on soy sauce. If you shorten your rice with a spoonful of this spice, you simply increase the sodium by 600 mg.

What's the deal with salt? Excessive intake of this mineral is associated with persistent hypertension. An example was found with more than 4,000 adults, and these people ate high degrees of sodium and had regular additions to improve their hypertension that increased their consumption. Next time you go to the grocery store, look for low sodium soy sauce and be optimistic about maintaining your ingredient dimension under control.

10. Maple Syrup

Derived from the bark of maple trees, maple syrup is about 100% sugar. The syrup carries sucrose, which is damaged in glucose and fructose. While too much glucose may cause spikes in blood sugar, research suggests that too many tons of fructose may increase your risk for non-alcoholic fatty liver disease.

Do not fall for claims that a particular brand of maple syrup is sugar-free. According to Eat This, Not That !, a sugar-free capacity product can contain less than 0.5 grams of sugar per serving. A typical serving of maple syrup is one tablespoon - however, most of us measure how good syrup we put on our pancakes, to be honest. And real maple syrup cannot be reduced to sugar. If you want some candy with your pancakes, try using light molasses or whipped cream instead of sugar-filled syrup.

11. Guacamole

According to Authority Nutrition, avocado is an excellent source of nutritious fat in itself. But the amount of food a traditional man or woman can eat sitting in a room is problematic. It is almost impossible just to dip a chip in a bowl of guac and walk away, and you know about it. Most Gokamol recipes call for two to three whole avocados, providing up to a ton as nine full avocado servings. A hundred grams of avocado contains about 15 grams of fat. They may contain healthy fats, but many nutrients of any kind can still be harmful.

Making your guacamole returned to sodium is an excellent first step. You can make very little of what the traditional recipe says, which dramatically reduces your eating chances.

12. Sour Cream

Your favorite baked potato accessory is a lot less than you think. Full-fat buttercream contains 3 grams of saturated fat per teaspoon. There is also about 30 energy per serving, which probably won't be visible anymore - unless you consider how small a small spoon is, of course - your thumb, from knuckles to tip, a tablespoon. Measurement. Your Wendy's Ripe Potato brings a full packet of Sour Cream, which is no longer just the size of a thumb.

Instead of sour cream, use plain Greek yogurt as a spice. Unlike bitter cream, Greek yogurt is, according to Greatest, full of protein and probiotics. The texture and style are incredibly comparable when used as toppings.

13. Honey Mustard

You can opt for honey mustard over mustard every day for the sweetness it brings, but if you are shopping for it, you are at a considerable disadvantage. A honey mustard bottle of sweet baby ray contains sugar, soybean oil, egg yolk, and yellow dye. Like many processed sauces, more and more ingredients are not there to maintain the product and prolong its shelf life. However, lookup dyes such as yellow five would likely be carcinogenic. It may be an animal study, but it is hardly encouraging.

Homemade honey is simple to make mustard and a fantastic, very healthy thing you can buy in a jar or bottle. All you need is honey, mustard, cayenne pepper, and a little bit of vinegar. No yellow pigment or various additives, and tastes much better.

14. Tartar Sauce

The seafood is unbelievable, with a bit more flavor. Tartar sauce may no longer be an excellent way to get that eclectic taste. Two tablespoons of McCormick brand tartar sauce contain three grams of sugar, one hundred and forty calories, 14 grams of fat, and one hundred and ninety milligrams of sodium. Ingredients include high fructose corn syrup, lemon juice concentrate, and herbal flavor.

Food labels are notorious for their natural phrases, such as "natural flavor." As David Andrews, Ph.D., tells life through the Daily Burn, natural flavors are nothing more than chemicals extracted from whole foods and delivered to processed ingredients in a laboratory. Grinding fish with herbs and olive oil is a very healthy way to eat seafood.

15. Relief

For many people, a hot canine is not complete except for a crunchy, dill-infused overtopping. Unfortunately, the easiest sodium-per-serving counts on this list are in store-bought souvenirs.

Heinz Dill Relish has zero calories, fat, or sugar listed on its vitamin label. However, 1 tbsp is equivalent to 230 mg of sodium. This is usually due to the excessive vinegar and salt content of the condenser.

You will additionally find preservatives, herbal flavors, and yellow dye five on this label - enough to inform you that adding a little crunch to your hot dog may no longer be a fair idea after all. Foods high in preservatives and various additives are associated with achieving viable weight gain and obesity.

You can bring your appreciation to the household level, using fresh dill, cucumbers, vinegar, onions, and other nutritious ingredients while keeping waste food additives off. Or you can altogether bypass the taste and try to revel in your cookout.

1 Buy a nonstick pan

Cooking from scratch is one of the most luxurious approaches for retailers on calories. However, by paying interest in what you are cooking, you can reduce even more without problems. Cooking with oils can add hundreds of calories to a meal (with most oils having 120 calories per tablespoon of pills), in addition to contributing significantly to its flavor regularly. To cut down on wasted calories, invest in a non-stick pan that requires very little oil or, in some cases, none at all. two

2 Recreate your favorite behavior

Making homemade versions of your favorite treats can help you shop on calories without compromising on taste. By doing your goodies, you are in charge of the things that go into them and can swap components in addition to reducing calorie content. For example, try changing sugar for agave nectar (which is sweeter than sugar, so you want less), replacing cream with evaporated milk or yogurt, and adding low-fat coconut to your favorite curry—use of milk. Cooking also burns more calories than opening the packet, making it a top-notch calorie-saving method. two

3 Spice up your food

If you are looking to reduce the number of calories in your food, then using more spices, herbs, and chilies can help. Incorporating herbs and seasonings into your foods can add extra flavor to your food and provide a kick to your food, adding any more calories. As a distributed bonus, chili peppers and spices such as cinnamon, cayenne, black pepper, and ginger can simply promote weight loss, supporting you to burn off any super flake energy consumption. two

4 Discard spices

If you consider yourself a healthy eater, yet you cannot lose more and more of these pounds, it may be time to reflect on your food and what you are doing. Is. Oily and sugary dressings, dips, and sauces can, in any other case, add a relatively high amount of energy to healthy and low-calorie foods. Avoid these peeled calories by opting for small amounts of low-calorie spices such as balsamic vinegar, salsa, or brown mustard, or skip these extras altogether.

5 Buy small plates

While you can only eat three meals every day, many of us have gotten into the habit of eating a great deal, just what we need, which means that you should eat six or more famous servings each day as many of us feel compelled to eat portions on a large scale, undoubtedly since they are there, our self in facing temptation through buying only small amounts of their favorite treats. Help - even if they seem like an accurate value for money! Also, try swapping your plates, bowls, and glasses for younger people, which will help you manage your serving sizes. two

6 Chew more slowly

It usually takes a minimum of 20 minutes for your body to record feelings of fullness, which means that the more you consume your food, the more you will feel compelled to finish before you experience it. Research results published in the American Journal of Clinical Nutrition showed that people who chew every forty times eat about 12 percent less energy than those who chewed only 15 times, so every bite helps reduce calories after Try to take your time. two

7 Cut back on liquid calories

While many of us pay interest for what we eat, we often bounce these energies into liquid form. However, these may want to add a more considerable amount of your daily total. While alcohol is the primary liquid calorie culprit, soft drinks, fruit juice, smoothies, and many hot beverages can also include the right size of calories and regular dietary value. To reduce your calorie consumption in addition to changing what you eat, try swapping a calorie-rich drink herbal tea or water. Alternatively, the choice of milky drinks for skinned variations and fizzy drinks for diluted fruit juices with sparkling water. two

8 Get more sleep

Research suggests that getting extra sleep can be a trick in an increasingly difficult way to get back to your calorie intake. A Columbia University study has found that when humans are deprived of sleep, they eat about 300 energy a day when they get enough rest. The idea that this is because lack of sleep stimulates the formation of our starvation hormone,

Ghrelin, while also decreasing the degree of leptin, the hormone that makes you feel full.

9 Choose filling foods

If you want to eat less energy but still feel full, you need to be smart with your food choices. Opt for filling in additional materials in protein and fiber, which can help you make complete sense in the long run). Also, choose 'heavy' foods, which will fill you up after consuming lots of calories. Experts at the University of Sydney have primarily developed a 'veracity index' of how long you will be exhausted by feeling hungry, and of potatoes, fish, oats, apples and oranges, whole pasta, beef, beans, grapes Recognized as the most filling material. , Bread, and popcorn. two

10 Pay attention to your food

Many of us eat calories unnecessarily honestly since we are not paying attention to what we are eating; according to the lookup findings posted in the British Journal of Nutrition, eating while distracted may cause you to pass signals to your body that you have had enough, mainly because you will eat extra for yourself. To reduce your calorie intake, try to consume on the table, and research to fully taste your food, then in front of a TV or laptop screen.

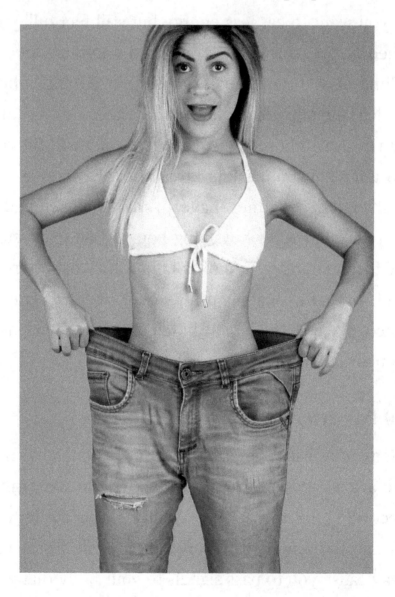

CHAPTER 3
Anticipate temptation

In a new study, individuals predicting the temptation to act unethically were less likely to supply in that temptation, in contrast to those who no longer had a chance to proceed.

The findings, published in the journal Personality and Social Psychology Bulletin, may explain why some humans commit suicide rather than moral resistance.

"People often believe that bad humans do horrific cases and that top humans do the right thing, and that unethical conduct comes only to character," lead research author Oliver Sheldon, Ph.D.

"But most humans sometimes behave dishonestly, and often, it may have more to do with the extra scenario and how a human sees his immoral conduct than character."

In a series of experiments, contributors conducted for future inducements were less likely than those who did not prepare for these preparations. These members were less likely to endorse unethical behavior that supplied non-permanent satisfaction, such as stealing office components or illegally downloading copyrighted material.

Sheldon, an assistant professor of organizational conduct at Rutgers University, said, "Self-control, or the lack thereof, can be the one thing that explains why good humans sometimes do sinister things."

In one experiment, 196 business-school students are divided into pairs: a man or woman was once a "buyer" and "seller" of various ancient houses. Before the talking exercise, 1/2 of the group noted moral temptations; He wrote about a time in his life when bending the rules was useful, at least in the short term, while the control crew wrote about a time when back-up graphs helped.

Agents were told that the property should only be offered to a buyer who would keep the ancient properties and no longer ruin them for new development. However, the shopkeepers were instructed that their consumers planned to demolish the properties and build a high-rise hotel, although they were ordered to hide that record from the seller.

The findings confirmed that more than two-thirds of consumers (67 percent) in the management team lied about hotel plans to close the deal, compared to fewer than half (45 percent) of buyers who Were reminded of the temptation in writing practice.

The temptation of temptation can only help; however, if a human believes that an immoral act has the potential to damage their self-image, integrity, or reputation.

In a second scan with seventy-five university students, members were placed to flip a coin, labeled as "SHORT" or "LONG," to determine if they were spelled and Proof of short or long passage of textual content for grammatical errors.

Individuals have been bitten by two agencies that completed the same writing practice as the first test (recalling unethical behavior or back-up planning).

Additionally, half of the individuals were told that a person's values, lifestyle goals, and character were stable, while the other group was informed that these symptoms could be dramatically altered within a few months. This data impacted whether members would see their behavior in work as consistent or who they would be in the future.

Participants who were encouraged to follow the temptation and were instructed that their conduct was stable with their future selves were honest: they suggested that small coins were unlikely to burst.

On the other hand, those who were no longer motivated to rely on temptation and believed that their conduct was inconsistent with their future selves had the additional possibility of lying about the extent of the small coin's fluctuations. So they have to do very little work.

Suppose a person wishes to abstain from unethical behavior. In that case, it may help count the possible temptations and reflect on the trick as to how acting on these temptations applies to long-term goals or beliefs about one's morality.

"Also, if a human is located outside, you may not be concerned about being caught or your popularity, but you may be concerned about your very own moral self-image," Sheldon said.

"Considering such issues, entering a person's skeptically enticing circumstances can help a human face the temptation to behave unilaterally."

"People often think that horrible people do terrible things and that top human beings do good work, and that unethical conduct comes only to the character," says lead looking writer Oliver Sheldon, Ph.D. "But most humans sometimes behave dishonestly, and often, this may be more to do with the landscape and how humans view their immoral conduct than character."

In a sequence of experiments, individuals who anticipated the temptation to act unethically were much less likely to behave unethically, which was not related to these people. These participants probably did little to advocate unethical behavior that provided temporary benefits, such as stealing office elements or illegally downloading copyrighted material. This was once posted online in the Personality and Social Psychology Bulletin on 22 May 2015.

Sheldon, an assistant professor of organizational conduct at Rutgers University, says, "Self-control, or the lack thereof, may be the one thing that explains why proper humans do terrible things."

In one experiment, 196 business-school college students were divided as consumers or sellers of some historic homes. Before the negotiation exercise, half the people in the group were reminded of moral temptations; He wrote about a time in his life when bending the regulations was once useful, at least in the short term, while the management team wrote about a time when back-up sketches helped.

Dealers have been informed that the property is offered only to a customer who will preserve the historic residences and no longer ruin them for new development.

However, shopkeepers were told that their customers planned to demolish the dwellings and build a high-rise hotel, but they were ordered to hide that record from the seller.

More than two-thirds of buyers (67 percent) in the manipulating team lie about hotel plans, so they may want to close the deal, compared to less than half (45 percent) of consumers who Were reminded of the temptation—writing practice.

However, a retaliation to temptation may also help if people identify an immoral act as an ability to jeopardize their self-image, integrity, or reputation. In a second experiment with seventy-five university students, individuals were placed to flip a coin, once labeled as "SHORT" or "LONG," to determine if they had Evidence for a quick or long passage of text for spelling and grammatical errors. Individuals were divided into two companies that performed the same writing workout as the first experiment (recalling unethical behavior or a back-up plan). Also, half of the participants have been instructed that an individual's values, lifestyle goals, and personality are stable, while the other crew was informed that these traits might be fundamentally optional even within a few months.

This record is used to influence whether contributors will have to watch their conduct in the project statically, which will happen to them in the future.

Participants who were influenced to rely on temptation and who regularized their behavior with their future have been sincere: they reported brief coin flaps that were not taking off by chance.

However, people who did not influence to expect temptation and who believed that their behavior was inconsistent with their future selves were probably in addition to lying about the quick coin flip's extent so that they have to work less.

People may also be more likely to interact in unethical behavior if they believe that the act is an autocratic phenomenon. In an online scan with 161 participants, humans have been given less inclination to help unethical conduct in six locations of job situations if they anticipate temptation through writing practice and all six scenarios in a single Considered at the bar, rather than expecting attraction and thought. They were considered every situation on a separate PC screen. The procedures depleted workplace supplies, calling when sick, only working slowly when tired, and deliberately staying away from extra tasks.

"Unethical conduct also cannot be efficient because there is something that one wishes to oppose if a man believes it to be socially ideal or no longer replicates his moral self-image," Sheldon says. "People often compile their experiences of seduction, which makes it very easy for them to rationalize behavior. They can say, 'Just because I once took domestic elements for office for personal use, It does not mean that I am a thief. '"

If humans favor abstaining from unethical behavior, it may help to anticipate situations in which they would be tempted and reflect the idea that the act of such inducement would be long-term about their morality, how it fits with wishes or beliefs.

"You may not be concerned about being caught or your popularity if people are located outside, but you will probably be concerned about your moral self-image," Sheldon says. "Keeping such concerns in mind that a person enters potentially enticing situations can help a human face the temptation to behave unethically."

Similar signs can follow for employers, Sheldon says. For example, a manager should meet with e-mail personnel before the workday to warn them against the temptation to increase travel expenses.

Reminders about the upcoming inducement can help protect the company's bottom line, especially if personnel see the temptation to increase travel costs as they will encounter many times in the future.

Ethical dilemmas quickly create the strength of mind enmity between pursuing the long-term advantages of behaving dishonestly and dating honesty.

Therefore, elements facilitating willpower for various goals (e.g., fitness and financial) should also promote ethical behavior.

In 4 studies, we find support for this possibility.

In particular, we find that solely under stipend that facilitates the identification of battles - including considering multiple options simultaneously (i.e., a more extensive decision frame) and excessive connectivity for future selves Relates to - expects a temptation behave honestly to promote honesty. We demonstrate these interaction patterns between identity and attraction anticipation of fighting in negotiation situations (Study 1), laboratory duties (Study 2), and ethical dilemmas in the workplace (Studies 3–4).

We conclude that there are two fundamental preconditions for coping with a will and making a proper choice to witness a temptation.

Although most societies care deeply about having a moral self-image and moral reputation, one only needs to see reports about tax fraud, bribery, steroid use, and academic misconduct that Is unethical behavior on a Large scale. Although a part of such action is moderately minor (Mazar, Amir, & Ariely, 2008), overall, even little every day can cause social and monetary damage. Currently, a long-repeated ethics violation has led to an appreciation of public confidence in sports activities and politics (Davis & Capello, 2013; JA, 2010), while the latest Association of Certified Fraud Examiners (ACFE; 2012) indicates the document; Most companies lose about 5% of annual revenue due to unethical behavior.

What does it tell when human commits suicide versus coping with morality-temptations? Although earlier work in behavioral ethics points to several elements that motivate humans to fail to behave ethically, regardless of their morality (Bazerman & Gino, 2012), the strength of mind also adverts behavior. May play an indispensable position in (Barnes, Schaubroeck, Huth, & Ghumman, 2011; Gino, Schweitzer, Mead, & Aireli, 2011; Mead,

Bumister, Gino, Schweitzer, & Arelli, 2009; Monin, Pidge Zija, and Beer; 2007; Tenbrunel, Diekmann, Wade- Wade Benzoni, & Bazerman, 2010). Ethical dilemmas create conflict strengths, presenting selection makers with a choice between pursuing a direction of action that gives short-term gains and others that show more long-term benefits.

Therefore, face-tors that help likers effectively navigate such conflicts across different domains (e.g., health, finance) require intelligent results to make more ethical decisions. It occurs. In the current research, we empirically test this opportunity, whether recognizing conflict and waiting for temptation are the two necessary conditions for making the moral choice.

Intra-psychic problems are ubiquitous and may have a student's choice of whether to watch TV, find out about upcoming exams, or choose a health-conscious dinner, but it's bland but tasty over nutritious options, But unhealthy penetration is for.

Because humans often internalize the past of others as their long-term personal interests, they may additionally encounter such conflicts in interpersonal domains, such as the finding that repeated encounters (Sheldon And Fischbeck) to cooperate or not (2011) or to have antisocial behavior towards others in close relationships (Buyukcan-Tetik, Finkenauer, Kuppens, & Vohs, 2013; Finkel & Campbell, 2001). Directly, there are many ethical dilemmas, especially whether or not they are involved. Be honest, create a similar problem (Monin et al., 2007). Specifically, such difficulties typically occur between existing behavior makers with a willingness to behave both unethically to achieve what they choose at the moment (e.g., dis- for example gains. Honesty) or behaving more morally (i.e., certainly toward others to maintain. A moral self-image, self-integrity, and the extent that their choice is public A are that honest popularity, and social acceptance goes on at length. Consistent with this observation, the previous lookup has shown that non-permanent impairment of self-control triggers through prior exertion of the strength of mind in an unrelated domain, Disc-Integrity (Barnes et al., 2011; Gino et al., 2011; Mead et al., 2009) and that low self-control is an essential factor in the production of criminal, antisocial conduct (Gottfredson and Hirschi, 1990). Note that ethical dilemmas can co-flick self-control. We recommend that two factors may interact and determine the likelihood of moral behavior: viewing multiple selection possibilities simultaneously, Which can promote recognition of the strength of conflict of mind, and increase the warning of temptation, which can encourage pre-exercise power of the mind, of impending conflicts. Face. To date, both of these factors have been extensively studied one by one (to fight intention, see Hoffman, Bomister, Forster, & Vohs, 2012; Raklin, 2000; Read, Loewenstein, & Rebin, 1999, for tempera-station; see Anticipation, Fischbach & Trope, 2005; Sheldon & Fischbach, 2011; Trope & Fischbach, 2000) and never in the context of ethical decision making.

Contraindications of these intercepted through mutual duality are rarely apparent to selection makers. Self-discipline conflicts are more routinely unclear as to how selectors incorporate temptation. For example, humans can no longer experience an immoral behavior in the first area as immoral-cal if they can body it as socially perfect (Tenbrunsel and Messick, 2004) or believe that This is the norm (i.e., everyone is doing it); Bandura, 1999; Reynolds, 2006). As an illustration, after entering doping, Lance Armstrong reported that he no longer thought he was being deceived because he saw a cycling field when all peak riders Use of tablets (Macur, 2013). For Armstrong, at least, doping no longer appears that the mind is a force of struggle.

Similarly, many petty "crimes," such as taking office resources for personal use or downloading content in addition to paying for copyright, may reflect the norm.

By no means does self-discipline induce conflict explicitly. One component that can influence self-discipline hostility is the structure of identity-on decisions; This is whether people collectively make a pair of choices associated with seduction in an inter-frame versus isolation (Myrseth & Fishbach, 2009); Read, et al., 1999). When likers encounter a given temptation, they may see it as a solo opportunity to act or one of the few similar temptations they will face over time (e.g., Nowadays they can eat one donut or 1 out of 20 donuts this month). Because the charge of the same inducement is negligible for regular long-term benefits, searching for conflict to look for possibilities simultaneously can also be kind of nil. The fixation results have been documented (Kahneman and Lovelow, 1993) in a wider variety-sous slender frame when evaluating the threat from view on intellectual bracketing (a simultaneous-order form of consumption decision). From (Simonson 1990), and thought-paradigm patterns in terms of addictions to single acts (Rachlin, 2000). In these studies, a broad bracket led to the practice of self-control. Those who adopt the body - interrelated vs. isolated, can similarly be formed through a phase of psychological con- madness, or the extent to which the choice maker views his / her non-thought. Public identities (e.g., state-of-the-art personality, temperament, values, beliefs, preferences, etc.) remain stable over time (Bartels & Rips, 2010). In this case, the less stability one sees in a person's non-public identity, the less likely it is to see a case or movements currently enticing as related or connected things that will entice someone in the future (Bartels & Urminsky) 2011). For example, suppose one's future will not feel an inducement to violate copyright laws independently. In that case, the selection may no longer be experienced as a will 22 holding the position, but rather, a separate violation As which no longer mirrors itself. Prior lookups have documented the association between perceived future and individual shifts in ethical choice making (Hershfield, Cohen, & Thompson, 2012). Building on the Hershfield et al.s (2012) work, we look at whether, more broadly, by looking at multiple decisions interconnected together, in a mutually related frame, hostility. Promotes identifying what else (as explained further) is an equally ethical move to the sale of looking ahead to temptation in advance.

Activating a person's thoughts about upcoming temptations (e.g., a donut) can determine the strength of will and the ten-term to act in a person's long-term self-interest (Fischbach, Freedman, and Kruglanski, 2003; Fishbeck & Trope; 2005).

It can put more pressure on people to overcome the—obstacles in chasing targets.

A simple reminder of the ensuing temptation may also prompt the person to indicate the desired response's strength that overcomes the temptation. Applied to an ethical context, presumably, makers who prefer equally to activate ideas about moral attractions should exercise greater self-control to have greater self-control when confronted with the resulting moral-ethical dilemma have to do?

A monetary mannequin of rational and arrogant behavior, which tells pre-makers that using a simple cost/benefit analysis for those who prefer, increases the expectation of moral temptations should make ethical behavior appear more expensive, leading to moral Decreases in the likelihood of performance (cf. Baker, 1968). However, work in the counteractive control idea (Fischbeck & Trope, 2007) introduces a strong counter-argument to this prediction, arguing that the moral dilemma certainly creates a self-con-troll conflict, temptation-related pictures should inspire people to behave more, not less morally. This is since selection makers may be prepared to pursue their preparations before repeating them at the tempera-station before such a temptation takes effect. For example, Fischbach and colleagues (2003) found that sub-teal priming participants used them to speculate about fatty foods (e.g., choke-oleate, cookies, chips) because of this file. Made more intentions to stop eating, and simply make more healthy food-related choices, unlike a con-troll crew (see also Zhang, Huang, & Broniarski, 2010).

Crucially, we do not argue that humans who suffer from temp- stations better follow their desires than those who do not. Instead, it is the hope of temptation (vs. no anticipation) for those who face temptation, which improves the counter-pattern by using the activation of self-control.

Taken together, we consequently recommend that when it comes to navigating moral ethics, whether humans will begin or not depends on whether they regard moral decadence-saints as interrelated Are, which helps them become aware of a problem.

To the extent that they do, a self-control workout must be done immediately to be morally over-behaved to raise warnings about an upcoming temptation (i.e., easy seduction-related thoughts). To the extent that they do not, waiting for attraction should not inspire efforts to respond to it.

We report the next four types of research that experimentally tested these propositions, creating a variety of experimental decision paradigm (interactive, personal, and vignette) and using a range of specific ethical dilemmas (e.g., to deceive Or not) in an interaction or performance of wrongdoing).

To manipulate developmental warnings, we have instigated temptation-related ideas, that is, whether members reflect efficient per-son or a general (faced by others) temptation before encountering these dilemmas. Huh.

To manipulate inter-lettered framing, we viewed participants as having their identity-relationships more or less stable (Study 2) or navigating multiple moral temptations versus them at different (unrelated) Was (mutually related; studies three and 4). Class 1: Resisting cheating in a conversation. In this preliminary study, we placed the participants' attention (and for this reason identification) as the strength of the mental conflict, which provided them with increasing persistence and two high, conscientious distinctions warning of an accurate moral inducement. In particular, participants are enrolled in a business enterprise negotiation direction and participated in a classification simulation stage. This sim-ovulation, which involved a buyer-seller real-estate transaction, only captures an ethical position for customers; To reach the agreed-upon moment, customers had to lie to the seller about their intended use of the property. Before negotiating, we observed consumers (through a previously unrelated pilot study) to recall the last time they encountered a temptation or recall a neutral past event. Our necessary structured measures are aimed at buyers' honesty (or lack thereof) in negotiations. We imagined that recalling times when one encounters a temptation (vs. neutral event) will limit buyers' deception. The specific rule for predefined pattern sizes was 20 or more per cell once for laboratory studies (Simmons, Nelson, and Simonotion). 2011, recommendation) and double that number-ber for classroom-based and on-line courses, which is characterized by accelerated noise that regularly indicates later con-texts. Because this color shows only about half of the pattern used in the analysis, a pattern dimension of about a hundred and sixty was pre-finished. To achieve this, we invited all 226 Masters-level Business School College students to all sections of the Conversation Guidelines to find out about the part of their curriculum. A total of 196 individuals set up invitations (67 women). Given that a member (buyer) of every interaction as a whole was undoubtedly faced with an ethical dilemma, and that for this reason, all analyzes are entirely focused on the integrity of this member, for all analyzes, Our overwhelming sample was 98. The currently existing study used a temptation Vs. Neutral prime, between-subject design. Buyer assigned to participants

The role garnered one of two forms of a volatile "pilot study" on retrospective perception, believed to aid the class teaching assistant with her dissertation for Candy.

In one version (temptation-prime condition), these members were brought up to remember and write about a time in their lives "when bending the rules were useful, at least in brief times.

" In an alternate version (neutral) -prime situation), they are triggered to recall and write about a time in their lives "when a contingency (i.e., back-up) graph was useful.

" Common recollection in the inducement-prime condition provides a blanket for prior cases of petty bribery.

Work-related shortcuts, and exploiting flaws in organization policy.

The neutral-prime state requires a back-up to graduate college in recruitment, so that they may have to seek their choice or adopt someone because of not getting their desired job.

To help with Cowl's story, the contributors' role also completed this experimental study, albeit only in the neutral-predominant version. All contributors were given 1 hour to play the role of "Bullard houses."

DRRC], 2008), a buyer-seller real estate transaction involving the sale of a historical set of homes. In this simulation, individuals interacted as the buyer's agent ("buyer") or the seller's agent ("seller").

This simulation was chosen because it gives negotiators many options for customers to respond to the ethical dilemma (Carey, Kennedy, & Van Zant, 2014).

Sellers have been steering solely to promote the property to only one consumer who will prioritize its modern-day structure and, preferably, its residential purpose ("You should certainly ensure that homes are destroyed" Will not be done; maximizing the sales charge is essential only later.

"The above interests are satisfied").

The buyer, whose education material presents some clues as to the seller's interests, was prohibited from disclosing on any occasion, whose patrons meant to build an industrial high-rise resort catering for tourists and convention visitors Was inconsistent with the pastime of vendors.

"Your customer has no longer recommended you under any circumstances use the website"). However, at no point were buyers forced to lie. Eliminate the barriers imposed by their own customer's path, as simple cognizance of the seller's past (and the subsequent moral conflict they face), the shopkeepers encountered while walking into this conversation. Whether or not it is accurate or complete vs.

dishonest with marketers about their client's intended use of the property. Because deception leads to powerful temptation in every conversation (cf. Gino & Shea, 2012), and because participants knew that they would negotiate different instances in later weeks as a part of their course, we hypothesize that Buyers decided in an interrelated frame. Buyers who demonstrate complete honesty can inform the seller that they were barred from disclosing the alleged use of the property, although doing so would almost raise suspicion and create an impasse.

Alternatively, different levels of dishonesty can be used; Buyers can declare that they were unaware of their customer's intended use, focusing on ambiguous phrases such as residential (although a motel "people of homes," it is temporary and has special zoning compared to long-stay accommodations Require), or explicitly lie with the aid of the claim, claiming that their client has the property to follow the seller (i.e., their Roman format should bring in regular use with maintaining).

After their negotiation, each gamer completed a post-negotiation questionnaire assessing buyers' deception in the present study. Our first and foremost measure was once whether or not individuals suggested accomplishing a deal in their negotiation. As indicated above, the only way shoppers and agents should attain a deal was once if the client misled the seller about their intended use of the property as soon as purchased. To complement this outcome-based measure, we likewise queried buyers directly about how misleading they were, asking them whether or not they know the vendor that the property would be developed for industrial use (4-point scale, with higher numbers indicating greater dishonesty; 0 = Yes; 1 = I did now not specify; 2 = Not exactly. Part commercial, section residential; 3 = No. Non-commercial use only). To take a look at that buyers' money owed matched those of their vendor counterparts, we requested agents a model of this identical direct question ("Did you be aware of whether or not the property would be developed for commercial use?"), using the identical scale, albeit tailored to match their version of the question. Results and discussion analyzed the proportion of buyer-seller dyads that reached an agreement. We dealt with achieving a deal in this case as proof that the customer involved had been dishonest with the seller. As predicted, a smaller proportion of dyads in which the purchaser had been primed with temptation (45%) reached offers than did dyads with a neutrally primed client (67%), $\chi2(1, N = 98)$ = 5.01, p = .04. Next, we analyzed responses to our self-report measure of purchaser deception—the extent to which consumers informed sell-ers that the property would be developed for business use (i.e., their true purpose). Supplementing our first analysis, consumers primed with temptation stated less deception about the commercial usage to which they planned to put the property (M = 1.14, SD = 0.79) than did neutrally primed customers (M = 1.51, SD = 0.98), t(96) = −2.04, p = .04, $\eta p2$ = .04, 95% CI = [−0.73, −0.10]. Incidentally, this was once proven by using their seller counterparts, who have been less possibly to file that they had been deceived (M = 1.00, SD = 1.06) than were vendor counterparts of neutrally primed buyers (M = 1.49, SD = 1.02),

$t(96) = -2.33$, $p = .02$, $\eta p2 = .05$, 95% CI = $[-0.91,$ $-0.07]$.

These findings supply initial support for our hypothesis that reminding humans of temptations before encountering an ethical self-control conflict leads them to counteract the predicted impact on ethical temptation and behave more ethically. Hence, we report the first proof for counter-active to manipulate in the ethical domain.

Study 2: Anticipated Temptation Promotes Ethical Performance for the Psychologically ConnectedTo check whether or not human beings solely exercise strength of will and behave more ethically in response to temptations when they perceive the present state of affairs in an interrelated frame (i.e., as associated to similar, future situations), in Study 2, we adapted a lab-based moral decision-making paradigm (Touré-Tillery & Fishbach, 2012; see Batson, Thompson, Seuferling, Whitney, &amp additionally; Strongman, 1999). In this task, participants first accomplished identical temptation-priming manipulation as used in Study 1. Also, we manipulated one component in all likelihood to affect whether they would discover a, as a result, encountered moral predicament as related to similar, future decisions they would possibly confront (i.e., adopt an interrelated frame): their degree of psychological connectedness to their future selves (Bartels & Rips, 2010). Participants then completed some computer-based proofreading tasks. Individuals confronted an ethical dilemma: supply into the temptation to assign oneself to brief versions of the undertaking (which entailed much less work) or give oneself to whatever task versions one's coin flips befell to indicate. We predicted that solely those who felt strongly psychologically connected to their future self would behave greater truly in response to primed temptation. To permit an initial test of whether the strength of mind operations would explain this anticipated interplay effect, we also had participants document whether or not they skilled a self-discipline conflict in the study.ParticipantsBased on prior work (Bartels & Urminsky, 2011), we predicted our psychological-connectedness manipulation would exhibit a moderate measurement effect.

Consequently, a sample size of eighty individuals was once predetermined. To obtain this, we invited 100 undergraduates from an organizational behavior direction to participate for more excellent credit, and seventy-six (38 female) ultimately opted to do so. One participant failed to complete one of the experimental manipulations, leaving a remaining sample of seventy-five participants.

ProcedureThe existing find out about used a 2 (prime: temptation or neutral) × 2 (psychological connectedness: high or low) between-subjects design. Participants performed the computerized proof-reading assignment in non-public cubicles and unmonitored.

Participants learned that the mission assessed "reading comprehension, verbal skills, and interest to detail for exclusive sorts of passages with some writing contexts, styles, and lengths.

" Their assignment would be to proofread eight extraordinary passages overlaying some subjects and containing spelling, grammatical, and different kinds of errors in completing it.

Participants further examine that they would proofread either a short version (containing two errors) or an extended version (containing ten errors) for every ride.

For the experiment, lengthy and brief passages had to be assigned randomly. Therefore, before each course, they would be precipitated to flip a coin to decide which version to read. For this purpose, we gave every participant their cash, labeled "SHORT" on one aspect, and "LONG" on the other. After each coin flip, they have been prompted to enter the consequences of their flip into the computer earlier than transferring on to proofread the authentic paragraph

Using this paradigm, we created incentives for claiming that the coin landed on SHORT (i.e., the favorable outcome): analyzing a shorter passage, discovering fewer errors, and completing the experiment faster.

This feature, in turn, created an ethical catch 22 situation for participants.

We labeled every coin to restriction ambiguity, confusion (honest mistakes), or self-deception that should happen when human beings first flip the coin and then try to determine the which means of the consequence (e.g., whether "heads" skill they ought to examine the short or lengthy passage; see Batson, Kobrynowicz, Dinnerstein, Kampf, &amp additionally; Wilson, 1997; Batson et al., 1999).

Immediately after learning about the above task, but before assignment it, individuals performed two experimental manipulations, framed as unrelated pilot studies for two one of a kind researchers.

First, members done the equal temptation-priming manipulation as in Study 1, recall-ing and writing about both a time in their lifestyles when bending the regulations was useful, at least in the quick run (temptation-prime condition) or a time in their life when having a contingency (i.e., back-up) design was once beneficial (neutral-prime condition). Second, participants accomplished a manipulation of psychological connectedness tailored from Bartels and Urminsky (2011) meant to affect whether they recognized the upcoming undertaking as posing a strength of mind conflict. Specifically, individuals assigned to the high psychological-connectedness condition examine a quick description of recent lookup and scientific information suggesting that one's non-public identification is some distance extra steady than most human beings understand (e.g., "the traits that make you the person you are right now—your personality, temperament, primary likes and dislikes, beliefs, values, ambitions, lifestyles goals, and ideals—are established early in existence and constant via the give up of youth . . ."). Participants assigned to the low psychological-connected-ness condition, on the other hand, examine how recent research and information cautioned that one's private identification is some distance much less steady than most humans realise (e.g., "the vital traits that make you the man or woman you are proper now—your personality, temperament, principal likes and dislikes, beliefs, values, ambitions, lifestyles, goals, and ideals—are in all likelihood to exchange radically, even over the route of a few months . . .”). To make sure comprehension, members wrote a one-sentence precis of the passage they read. Finally, individuals performed the primary proofreading task and crammed out a post-task questionnaire.

Are you ready to face temptations? Two, they will come - there is no question. Two, we no longer know when or where, although you will be tempted if you are a human being. The penalty of not being ready now can be frightening. Think of the person who is drawn to watch porn or the anger building inside you that should burst at any moment. Give it something small or big - we want to be ready for temptation in our lives.

Some humans have evolved to recognize their moments of vulnerability. They have kept watch guards safe from temptation. This is one of the purposes we have for internet filtering. Two, but what if the attraction does not begin at excellent moments? The two temptations will often start in the routine of life. Then they can build up to be some extraordinary thing.

This is the state of affairs Jesus and his disciples find themselves in Luke 22: 39–46.

The Usual Place

At this moment toward the struggle of Jesus' life, he brings his disciples from the upper chamber, and they made their way to Mount Olives. The Bible uses an interesting phrase to describe the region - "He went out and made his way as usual ..."

This was a regular practice for Jesus. The Mount of Olives is the place they used to visit often. There are two familiar places where Jesus teaches his disciples to anticipate temptation.

Most of the people I understand have normal life activities. When you're in your routine, you can reach a point where you're not just questioning - you're just repeating the same trick over and over. Two, I have been riding the same route to work for twenty years. Two days make me wonder how I got there because I just go through the events and don't even think. Sometimes, I take a seat and watch TV as a routine. Two, I, too, am not paying much attention to what I am doing.

When we get caught up in the giddiness of our routine, we can lose sharpness, and this is where Satan can strike with temptation. This may be what was happening to Jesus' disciples. Two, they are going back to the equal area as usual. But this time, Jesus tries to warn them that temptation may also be, and they need to be ready.

Jesus' Method for Preparing for Temptation

You can also have all kinds of strategies and techniques to help deal with temptations. There may be two when you count to 10 feelings angry; there is a pure filter or an accountability partner. All these things are appropriate and helpful, but they are no longer what Jesus teaches his disciples here.

Jesus has an essential vision for his disciples - prayer. Two as they have been in their commonplace, he says, "Pray so that you do not fall in love."

How Prayer Helps Us Prepare for Temptation

Prayer helps us to be closer to God. Two Hearing her voice can help us see the temptation of too late.

Prayer helps us to shed light on the goodness of God. Temptations become much less attractive by seeing the personality and blessings of God. They pale in comparison to him.

Prayer reminds us that we are susceptible to temptation. We want God to protect us.

Prayer reminds us that we are not as strong as we believe we are. Two, we want God's help to say no to temptation.

John MacArthur put it this way, "We need to empty all the power of our spiritual glory, for all the overestimation of our strength, and pray for divine help." The two are not caught when the temptation hits with all their might, no longer praying. It helps wait for the one who prays. "

Jesus did not sleep

Jesus' disciples went into the common area and fell asleep - even though Jesus instructed them to pray because they did not fall into temptation. Jesus sees them lying there and repeats their command to pray once again.

Satanic is real. He wants you to spoil and rob you. Two, but he is additionally sly and deceitful. He will wait until you protect yourself. Two of us have a phase that always needs to be aware that temptation can come at any moment.

Thankfully, Jesus did not sleep that night. Two, he prayed - and he prayed hard! These prayers prepared him for the devastating betrayal and extreme exploitation he experienced with the temptations to move away from his identity and purpose.

Jesus prayed instead of sleeping. Two, because he remained devoted and devoted to his father, we are also likely to overcome temptation.

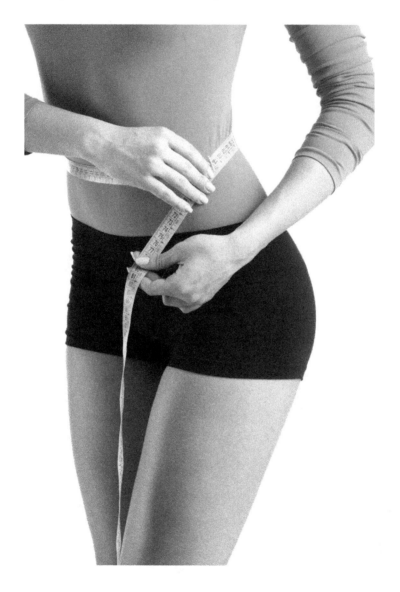

CPSIA information can be obtained
at www.ICGtesting.com
Printed in the USA
BVHW091240040521
606415BV00004B/871

9 781802 740196